I0426644

My Sudden Heart Attack

How I Recovered and Restored my Health through Weight Loss and Exercise

By

Edward Olsen

ISBN: 978-1-312-90957-1

Table of Contents

Chapter one
There's No Need to Worry About My Weight

When I was young, I thought I was invincible. I thought my health would never fail me and I would live to a ripe old age. I suppose it's not unusual for a young person to think that they are going to live forever and not give a thought about their future health. But I actually did think about it. I thought it through a little bit and figured that I would never have anything to worry about and that I really would live to a ripe old age and do just fine getting there. I thought this way because of what you might call my family heritage, or what most people would call "good genes." You see I thought I had really good genes. And actually, I suppose I did.

My paternal grandfather lived to be eighty two, and actually died of pneumonia in a hospital. I figured dying of pneumonia in a hospital didn't really count, so I thought I was okay there. My other grandfather did very well too as far as health issues go, so that was two for two in my mind.
My dad hadn't done so well but I wrote that off as a consequence of his lifestyle. He liked to drink beer and worked real hard all his life. So I figured that was what did him in.

When it comes to getting old and what is likely going to be a problem for you, most people figure it is either going to be cancer or heart disease. I figured I was set up pretty good on both of those issues because there was virtually no cancer in my family and no heart disease.

Looking back, now that I am much older, the view I had on both of those issues was a bit colored. I supposed I was looking through some rather optimistic sun glasses. There actually was some heart disease in my family, but not very much, and virtually no cancer. But from my point of view, I figured I was good.

I was sixteen when I got my first real job. I worked in a grocery store on the stocking crew. We were the guys who kept the shelves full of canned goods and whatever, all of the items the store sold. This was a rather large and very high volume grocery store, so it was hard work on freight days, when a semi-truck pulled up to the front door at about four o'clock in the morning and we unloaded it and stocked the shelves. We would go at it until about ten, when the store opened, and of course we had to have the store all cleaned up and ready to go by then.

My boss and two or three of the other guys liked to go to the gym to unwind after these tough mornings. They invited me to go along one day so I started going too. We drove across town to the Deseret Gym, which was owned by the Mormon Church. It was a nice gym, had two full size pools, racquetball courts, weight rooms, steam and sauna rooms. It was really a first class facility.

They had an elevated jogging track that ran around the periphery of one of the basketball courts. As I remember, it was fifteen or sixteen times around the track to make one mile. I remember the first time I tried to run it; my boss encouraged me to try to go for just a mile, and to take it easy and run slow. So I started running and ended up getting sick, and nearly puking up there on the track before I made the whole mile. But I kept going to the gym and running on that track, because I figured it help me in the long run. It didn't take very long until I could run the mile without much of a problem. I remember running that track many times while watching the guys play basketball games down on the court about twenty feet below.

That was how I got started running and from then on, as a form of exercise, when I did exercise, I enjoyed running the most. Now I wasn't really built for running. I had short legs and a stocky body, so I figured I would never be a track star, but I just liked to do it.

Later on when I was nineteen, I joined the navy and for exercise, I ran off and on as the situation would allow. I got into the nuclear power program and there, they were very concerned about any health problems you might have. I suppose it was because they were worried about lawsuits later on. So as candidates, we were all screened for health issues very closely. All the screening turned up no health issues on me, so that re-enforced my conviction that I was invincible and wasn't ever going to get any of the typical old age health problems that other people get when they get older.

One of the things they screened us for was diabetic tendency. They had a test for diabetic tolerance, as they called it, which involved taking a blood sample, checking the glucose level then having us drink this stuff that reminded me of Hawaiian punch base.

I am not sure if you can still buy Hawaiian punch, but it came in a half gallon bottle. You would mix about a cup full into a gallon of water to get your Hawaiian punch drink.

This stuff was thick, syrupy and it was sickening sweet, just like Hawaiian punch base. They made us drink a full cup of it. Then for the rest of the day we had to sit around and allow them to take blood samples every half hour or so to measure our glucose levels. This went on for about six hours and I passed the test with flying colors, further re-enforcing my belief of invincibility.

So it went for most of my younger years. I never seemed to have any health problems, certainly not cardiovascular. The only real problem I had, that might be classified as a health problem, I suppose, was keeping my weight under control. I never really considered that a health problem though, because during my younger years, I never really let it get out of control. Looking back though, I think that was mostly due to the navy and their attitude about being overweight. They didn't like it at all. It seemed that I was always on one weight control program or another just about the whole time I was in the navy and that was for thirteen years.

I remember that my weight hovered around 225 pounds or so all the time. Sometimes it was a bit less and of course, at times a bit more. The navy weight standard, at the time, said I should weigh no more than 183 pounds. They based that totally on how tall you were. I think there may have been allowances for whether you were big build or small. But I was six feet tall and that's the limit I had, 183 pounds. Now that I think about it, I don't think they really cared about your build, because I don't remember anyone ever being in trouble because they didn't weight enough. I think it was just that if you were six feet tall, you couldn't weigh any more than 183. And that was it.

The navy was rather pig headed about this. They said the reason for the concern was "military bearing." That really meant that they didn't want any fat looking navy guys. I suppose I can understand that, but even at the 225 or so, I really didn't look fat. I don't think I could have actually gotten down to 183, without looking like I was malnourished. But that didn't matter. It was one size fits all.

I struggled with my weight the whole time I was in the navy. It just didn't seem fair. I was no longer working on the freight crew, so I put on weight a lot easier. But I could see guys who were eating a lot more than me, who didn't seem to be gaining any weight, and I did. It just wasn't right. The professionals weren't any help either. I remember when I got accepted into a program that would lead to an officer's commission, there was a point when I had to make an appointment with a dietician so that she could tell me what I was doing wrong, not being able to get to my ideal weight limit of 183 pounds.

I remember meeting with this young lady who looked like she was fresh out of college. After the initial consultation, she asked me to write down everything I ate in the next few days and bring her the list, along with my weight readings. Well as the days passed, I can't remember how many days it was, but it was probably something like five I guess, I showed her the list and the weight readings, which didn't show a weight loss. I hadn't lost any weight at all. Well she looked over the list, assessing the calorie content I suppose, and she came to the conclusion that I was not writing everything down. There must be a few things that I had forgotten to write down, probably a lot of things. This just couldn't be, she told me in so many words. I could not be consuming only what was on this list and not lose weight.

I assured her that the list was true and it did contain everything I had eaten ……
everything!

Well rather than call me a liar, she called me a psychotic, saying that I must be eating other things and just not remembering it, wiping it from my memory because I was feeling so guilty, or something like that.

Well that ended my professional respect for dietitians, if I ever had any.

Then there was this guy in the class with us, who was eating way too much. Now he didn't look fat. As a matter of fact, he had very good military bearing, as the navy called it. But he would go to the chow hall and load his tray up until it was mounding over. He would do that three meals a day and not gain a pound. Well this caught the attention of someone important, and it wasn't long, after they watched him for a few days, until they got him a discharge. I suppose they thought they weren't going to be able to afford to feed him.

The reason I am telling you all this background about my struggle with weight is that when it comes to keeping your weight under control, you need to understand there are all kinds of people. We have all kinds of metabolism rates, and what works for one person may not work for another. So if you are trying to lose weight, it's not really good to compare what you eat to what someone else eats. We are all so different.

If you compare yourself to others, the danger you could run into is thinking that you can't lose weight, because you are doing what that other person is doing, but you're not losing weight, and then you give up because you think you just can't do it. But you really can.

If you have a weight problem, it does no good to compare yourself to someone who doesn't. And most of the time when you compare yourself to other people, that is exactly what you are doing. Most people who don't worry about what they eat, and naturally maintain a good body weight, don't have a weight problem. It is foolish to compare yourself to those people and try to draw any sort of productive conclusion. If you eat what they eat, of course you are going to gain weight. You have a weight problem and they don't. What else could you expect to happen?

On the other hand if you are looking for an excuse, that's a good one. But actually you can find all kinds of them. There's the thyroid problem. There's the slow metabolism problem. If your goal is to justify not even trying to stay fit and healthy, you can always find a reason like, "Oh it's not my fault I am fat, I have a thyroid problem."

But no matter how well you try to justify it to yourself, it is still only a lie. If you are really overweight, and you have that kind of mindset, and you don't try to take control of your eating habits, you are actually signing your own early death warrant. It will eventually catch up with you.

Chapter two
It Finally Caught up with Me.

When I finally got out of the navy I was really tired of constantly worrying about my weight and being continually hassled about it. I decided not to ever worry about it again. I was through with that. I was free.

Well it didn't take long, about six or seven months or so before I went from about 230 to 310 pounds. But I didn't worry about it. I was free and I refused to worry. Besides I had the "good genes," on my side so it really didn't matter, did it. Also, once I hit 310 pounds, it didn't seem to matter what I ate or how much. Once I hit that level, I stopped and stabilized there. So now life was much better, I thought. Gone was the constant worry about my weight. Life was good. I liked donuts. I liked chocolate milk. I ate them whenever I felt like it, with no ill effects. After all, I had good genes to protect me.

Well I went on this way for about twenty years and never gave it a thought. Of course I wasn't able to run anymore, but I really didn't care about that so much. I did occasionally do things like hiking and backpacking. I could do that, so I keep fairly active and didn't really notice that the effort it took to do those things was much more than it used to be. I guess that's because it crept up on me so slowly.

Well I was fifty five years old, and I was thinking I was relatively fit, and of course, blessed with good genes, so what could go wrong?

One day I bought a new evaporative air cooler for our house. This was one of those rather large, window mounted units. To install it, I needed to lift this thing up into place, into a rather tight spot. Because of the height and the tight spot, it was going to be rather difficult to do. I got my son to come over and help me. His job was to be on the inside of the house, where the cooler was to be mounted and once I had it lifted into place, secure it from the inside.

Well we did it. I lifted that big old swamp cooler into place, I was quite strong after all, but this thing was quite heavy. So I grabbed it and lifted it up until my arms were about head level. I held it there, in place until my son could get all the necessary brackets fastened so that it would stay. It didn't take very long. I only had to hold it for about thirty seconds or so, but it was heavy. I was greatly relieved when my son hollered from the inside, "Okay Dad. That's got it. You can let go now."

I think I was just about down to my last bit of stamina when he said that, so it was none too soon. I don't think I could have held it up much longer.

Well we did our high fives and then finished up installing it, buttoning everything up. I turned it on and it worked.

I didn't know it at the time, but I had just set into motion, a sequence of events that were going to kill in about twelve hours, had I not gotten to a hospital in time. They say there are typical warning signs that happen when you are having a heart attack. These are talked about in a lot of places so I won't go over them here. Rather, I will tell what happened to me. I will tell you what I felt. It wasn't really the same as the typical warning signs, probably because of my "good genes."

My "good genes," had helped me up to this point in life I believe, but this last time, my "good genes," betrayed me and almost killed me.

It was about five in the afternoon when we finished up. My son went home and after buttoning everything up, I settled in to watch some evening TV. I suppose it was about six or seven when I started to notice that I was feeling uncomfortable. That was about it. I wasn't in pain or anything like that. I just couldn't get comfortable sitting in my overstuffed easy chair.

I remember feeling something in my chest that I had never felt before, and I couldn't explain it. Now one thing in my favor was that I am an engineer, so I am accustomed to paying attention to detail, and if something was unexplainable, in a test for example, you don't chalk it up to, "oh well." You go and figure out what is happening.

Well, like I said, it didn't hurt. It was just odd and uncomfortable. I remember that it felt like a mild pressure, the kind you would feel along with a case of heartburn, if you'd eaten something that gave you a case of heartburn. The pressure feeling was there, but not the burn sensation. That is what was odd and caused me to take notice. What was happening? This was a new sensation that I had never felt before. But since it didn't hurt, I really didn't think of it as anything but odd at first.

Well as the evening went on, it didn't go away. I tried sitting up, I tried laying back. I got up and walked around, then sat down again. This feeling just wouldn't stop. Again, it didn't really hurt, it just felt odd, and I just could not get comfortable sitting in that chair.

Well, this went on for a couple more hours until it got to be about ten in the evening. It was time to get ready for bed. Because this odd feeling wouldn't go away, and it was something that I never felt before, I told my wife about it and said I should probably go to the hospital to have it checked out. I didn't think at that point that I was having a heart attack, but something odd was happening that I could not explain. So I didn't want to go to bed without having an explanation. Who knows, maybe it was a heart attack. So we got in the car and drove the twenty miles to the hospital. I drove, and I was still feeling fine, except for this strange feeling in my chest.

I remember when we pulled into the parking lot, next to the emergency room entrance. I still wasn't sure what to think. I didn't want to go in there for nothing. I noticed that the car was a bit low on gas and I got the idea to try one more thing first. I suggested that we go to a gas station, about five miles away, and get some gas. While there, I would go inside to buy some Pepto Bismol, and drink a bit down. Then we would drive back to the hospital, to see if that made it go away by the time we got back there to the hospital. That was the only test I could think of, that I could do on my own, that might help explain this. It would either explain it or it would once and for all tell me that it was definitely not some sort of indigestion, so I better get in there and figure it out.

Well I drove to the gas station. I went inside first and bought the Pepto Bismol. I opened it up while walking back to the car and took a big swig (after reading the dosage instructions of course). I got the gas, opened the hood to check the oil, and I was still feeling okay. But the Pepto Bismol didn't seem to be having any effect. The feeling was still there.

So I drove back to the hospital, parked in a good spot, not too far from the emergency room entrance. I was still feeling the same way, so we locked the car and I walked inside with my wife. There was a button just inside the door that was marked something like, "Push for Emergency." So I pushed it. It was a just a few seconds later that a couple of nurses came rushing around the corner, anxiously looking to see who had pushed the emergency button. Seeing me standing there with my wife, one of them said, in a rather urgent tone, "Is there something I can help you with?"

I answered, "Yes, I think I am having a heart attack."

I wasn't really sure what else to say, so I went for the big one. Either way that is what they should check for first. If it wasn't a heart attack, there would always be time to figure out what it really was.

Well they wasted no time in getting me into a wheel chair, wheeled me inside, asked me a few quick questions, then got me off to the emergency room.

Now you would think they would hook me up and do whatever they do to test for heart attacks and shortly afterward announce, that's what was happening, and get on with whatever they do for heart attacks. But that's not what happened.

Instead, they put me on a gurney, hooked me up and did their diagnostic stuff and got puzzled. Everything they measured was normal. So what was going on then? All of the electronic instruments were reading normal parameters. They did some chemical tests for heart attack chemical changes, and they turned out to show nothing was abnormal. My heart was still beating properly. My blood pressure was high, but that really didn't indicate anything of an emergency nature.

I remember looking at the clock in the little curtained off room they had me in. It was 11:30 PM. So here this all started, when I noticed something might be odd at about 6 or 7 PM and now, whatever was happening had been going on for about four hours or so, and they couldn't figure it out. The tests they did and the readings they were getting indicated this was not a heart attack. It was something else; but what?

Within an hour or so I began having chest pains. Now these chest pains were not like what I would have figured heart attack pains would be like. I had always figured it would be a pulsating sort of feeling. But it was not. The pain was steady and flat. It would start out at a low level and build up to a crescendo over a period of about a minute or two, then it would hang there at that intense, high level for about thirty seconds, then it would slowly subside over about the same time period and be gone for a while. When it hurt, it was very intense. It really hurt and seemed to fill my whole chest with pain. When it stopped, it would be gone for maybe a half hour or forty five minutes, then start up again.

They gave me a shot of morphine for the pain, but still my heart was beating normally, no abnormality to the rhythm at all. They ran some more chemical tests, and still there was nothing unusual. This went on all night. The pain kept coming and going, all the while, the tests and readings were all normal. I was having all the outward physical manifestations of a heart attack; the chest pains, the discomfort, yet none of the diagnostic devices or chemical testing could detect anything was wrong.

It went on like this until about 6:30 in the morning when a heart specialist, a cardiologist, came on duty for his normal work day. They called him to my curtained off little space in the emergency room, where we talked for a moment about what was happening with me. He was Russian, and had a slight Russian accent. He seemed like a very sharp fellow. As he took it all in and thought it over, he told me that there was no indication of a heart attack, but obviously something was going on, so he was going to have me admitted to the hospital where they would schedule some tests later on that morning to try and figure this out.

As he was about to leave, he took one last look at the electronic instrumentation that I was hooked up to, and it was then, at that moment, that my strong heart, with the good genes, finally gave up, and just couldn't do it anymore.

I remember he did a double take while looking at one of the displays, and then a second later it started beeping that tone of panic. "BEEP BEEP BEEP," it sounded off.

This Russian trained heart specialist apparently knew exactly what was happening at that moment. He immediately ordered the staff to get me into the operating room right now. I remember being quickly unhooked from all the instrumentation, and being wheeled out of the emergency room. I saw the changing ceiling panels and light fixtures go by as they pushed the gurney down the hall on its short journey to one of the operating rooms.

I was a bit groggy from all the pain killers and such they had given me, but I did not lose consciousness at all. It seemed like from the moment the gurney stopped moving, until they started telling me what was going to happen next, and then started doing it, it couldn't have been more than five minutes.

I was told I had a blockage in one of the major arteries of my heart and they were going to unblock it with an angioplasty procedure, then insert a "stent" in the artery to keep it open.

After the doctor, who was performing the procedure told me this, and started to inject a numbing medication in my groin area, I spoke up and said, "Well I guess it was a good thing I came back here. I could have had a heart attack."

When he heard this he stopped what he was doing, leaned my direction and looked me in the eye and said, "You did. You just had the big one."

Later on, as I was talking to him during the procedure, I mentioned that I had been thinking of going home earlier, telling him a little about getting the gasoline and all of that. He told me that he was certain I would not have made it back alive if I had done that.

Chapter three
What Happened to Me?

I did have a heart attack, that was true. But the question is why? What about my good genes? I never had any warning signs. There were never any chest pains before today. And I had, in the recent past, routinely done a lot of very physical things. This just came out of nowhere. How could that be?

Being an engineer, a geek, having the need to know how things work, I started asking a lot of questions of the doctors and of my cardiologist when he came to see me in the recovery room.

After thinking over what I learned in that conversation and my research since then, I am rather confident that what happened to me could potentially happen to anyone who is middle aged or more. There are no symptoms. In fact, what happened to me, as far as I can tell, is exactly what happened to the NBC News guy, Tim Russert. He died, on the job, in one of the sound proof recording studios at NBC while doing some preparation work for an upcoming news broadcast. He was only 58 years old. If you read about the details of what happened to him you will see the words, "ruptured cholesterol plaque," and where it happened, "left anterior descending artery."

That is exactly what happened to me, right down to the exact location in my heart. Mr. Russert had been to the doctor for a routine checkup not too long before this and even passed a stress test. That stress test should have provided some indication that he had a potential heart problem, right? So why didn't something show up? The answer to that question is somewhat disturbing if you trust in the infallibility of our medical system. This kind of thing has no symptoms. It really has no impending warning signs either.

Does that mean it's just something that's either going to happen or it's not? It's just a fresh roll of the dice, for each of us, every day? No, that's not necessarily what it means. If you have certain habits in your life, like I did, you can certainly make it have that meaning. From what I have learned, the potential may be there, but there is something that you can do to substantially decrease or actually increase the chances of this happening.

To help you understand the mechanism of this and what you can do about it, allow me to explain, in my geek, engineer, and hopefully simple way what actually happened to me.

Arteries are the blood vessels that carry the blood supply around your body, to feed all of your cells, wherever they may be. It's like this big garden hose that comes from your heart, (the pump) and branches off into thousands of little hoses to carry food all over your body.

Your heart is just a big muscle, and it needs a blood supply too and it can't get it from sucking it out of the blood that is flowing through it as it pumps. It has its own set of arteries that get their blood supply from the output side of the heart, that main big artery. Your heart has two or three (don't know the exact number) of its own main supply arteries (like the left anterior descending artery) that each branch off into many smaller and smaller sub-arteries that carry blood with food and oxygen to all parts of your heart to keep it fed. If one of these arteries gets plugged up, and blood stops flowing in that part of your heart, then that part of your heart begins to go to sleep and die. If a plug develops in one of the main arteries of your heart, that's very serious, because it means a large section of your heart, the entire section supplied by the plugged main artery, isn't getting blood anymore, so it starts to die. If that plugged artery isn't unplugged within about fifteen or twenty minutes, you will probably die.

So the question is how does an artery in your heart suddenly get plugged up like that? How does that happen? I always thought if your cholesterol levels were bad, you would be depositing a lot of plaque on the inside walls of your arteries and that's how they would get plugged up.

I am not a doctor, but I think that scenario is generally true. Serious heart problems do happen that way. But that's a long term process and as it happens over a period of time, you feel it happening, but the progression takes time; maybe several months or years. What happened to me was one minute I am just fine, and then within just a few hours, the artery is plugged. And I didn't even have high levels of plaque on the inside walls of my arteries. As a matter of fact, my doctor told me they figured my worst plaque levels were about twenty percent. Twenty percent is still rather low, and shouldn't have been any problem. So what did happen?

That's where the term, "ruptured cholesterol plaque," comes in. The way it was explained to me is that even if you have a relatively small amount of plaque, like the 20% or so that I have, it forms a coating that is something like a smooth lining on the inside wall of your arteries. Even though there is still plenty of room for good blood flow in an artery, if a crack should develop in any part of that lining on the inside wall of that artery, your body's own defense system goes into action, thinking that crack is an injury. We all know that if we get an injury like a small cut and we are bleeding, our blood begins to clot to plug it up to stop the bleeding. If you cut yourself, it doesn't take long for the bleeding to stop because your blood detects the injury and plugs up the hole.

Well if the plaque inside an artery cracks or "ruptures," your blood thinks an injury has occurred, and tries to plug up the hole. That is what will kill you, because in trying to plug up that hole, where the crack is, blood clots form and plug up the entire artery, cutting off the blood flow.

So now the question is, what causes the plaque to crack, or to "rupture?"

One thing that can do it is a sudden strenuous exertion that involves your upper body, perhaps lifting something very heavy. (That's what I was doing). But then again, sometimes it just happens. So the fruitful question really is; What can you do to prevent it from happening? What can you do to make the plaque that you already have less likely to rupture?

One answer might be to avoid doing any physical activity that might trigger a rupture. A better approach would be to try and "firm up" the plaque that you already have, so it's a bit more stable and less likely to rupture in the first place. But how can you do that?

Chapter four
What Do I Do Now?

When I was in the hospital room the next day, I had a good talk with my new cardiologist. All the lab test results were in for routine things they test for and we discussed them at length. The short story about those lab results is that I was a physiological basket case, and I had done it to myself over the years by not paying any attention to my health or fitness.

My glucose level when I arrived at the hospital the night before was about 460. For those of you who don't follow such things, it's a measure of how much sugar is in your blood. It would be normal to be around 100. It would be very bad if it was over 175. As you can see I was off the scale on that reading.

My A1C level was over 11. Again for those of you who might not know what that is, it's a measure of how many of your red blood cells are, in effect, "sugar coated". As they form, if your sugar levels are high, more red blood cells tend to form a sugar coating on them. And that sugar coating tends to stay in place as long as that cell is alive and well in your system. Red blood cells are always dying off and being replaced, so this is a good long term indication of how much sugar has been in your blood, on average, for the past thirty or so days. Normal is about 6.0 or 7.0. If you are above this it means you are probably a diabetic. As you can see, I was off the scale on this one too.

There were several other parameters that I won't bother you with, but they were all like this. They were all, for the most part, way out of bounds or off the scale.

So my good genes had been pulling me through the abuse I had been subjecting myself to for several years, until they just couldn't do it anymore. I was diabetic now, grossly overweight. I just had a heart attack. I was a physical wreck. The handwriting was on the wall, as they say.

In the conversation with my cardiologist, and from other research I had done, I came to the conclusion that the plaque on the inside walls of your arteries can get sort of spongy and delicate if your body chemistry is not good, because of high sugar levels for example, and being overweight. Lack of aerobic exercise is another contributing factor. Cholesterol readings out of whack, is still another contributing factor.

So to answer the question at the end of the previous chapter about what can be done to "firm up" the plaque that's already in your arteries; You get your body chemistry back in line and start doing aerobic exercise. The reason my plaque was so likely to rupture, as it did, and still was at that point in time, was simply that I was too fat and I never exercised.

Fixing up your body chemistry? That sounds rather daunting. Aerobic exercise? I hadn't done that in years. But if I could do that, I would be much better off and certainly not in imminent danger of another heart attack. I was only 55 years old at the time. I wasn't going to give up that easy. My attitude that my genes will protect me from all wrong had just been proven to me, by hard numbers, that it was a load of steaming Bull Shit! So if I was going do something that would prevent me from dying young, it was going to have to start with a change my attitude and lifestyle.

I was in the hospital for about five days. A nurse came in to see me on the second day to discuss how to eat properly, now that I was a diabetic. She showed me how to figure out dosage and how to use my insulin injection setup. She also put me on a diet while I was still in the hospital, where I was limited to something like 75 grams of carbohydrates per day.

Another nurse came in after that to discuss medications I would have to take to control my blood pressure. She also explained why high blood pressure was bad and all that sort of stuff.

Then another nurse came in to discuss cholesterol issues and why I needed to control that.

There were others that came in as well, to talk about all sorts of things that I needed to know. The truth is that I did know most of what they were trying to tell me. It was just that I always ignored it and didn't do what I should have been doing. I should have known better, but I was only fooling myself. There is so much information constantly out there, all around us, in commercials on TV, public service announcements, billboards and of course people just selling books about good health. There really is no excuse for not knowing this stuff. And actually, I did know it. I just chose to ignore it, thinking it wouldn't apply to me because I was special somehow. But I was forced to face the fact now that I was not really that special after all.

I was very fortunate that no heart damage had actually occurred, because when I actually had the "no kidding" classic heart attack, I was right there in the emergency room in the presence of a very good cardiologist, so very little time passed until I was treated, and proper blood flow was restored to my heart.

Well anyway, five days later I was discharged from the hospital, a diabetic, a heart attack patient, grossly overweight and in very poor physical condition. In addition to that, just about all of my chemistry readings were terrible; cholesterol, A1C, triglycerides, etc. I had been diagnosed with a bad case of high blood pressure as well. Just about anything you can think of that was a measure of how healthy you were, was way out of line.

So here I was, a basket case. Another heart attack was bound to happen if I didn't do something. But what should I do?

One thing I realized right away was that the way physicians tend to treat any of these conditions that I had was to give you some kind of medication for it. That's not bad, but in some ways, I figured that was not really going to cure me of anything. It was going to allow me to live with whatever I had wrong with me.

So I did more research on the root cause of all my problems. For example, my high blood pressure. I discovered most of that was likely hereditary, but my lifestyle had made it much worse. My father had high blood pressure too, and once I really looked into it, that was probably one of the big contributing factors to his early death. He was only 56 when he died. But does that mean I couldn't do anything about it, other than take drugs? No it didn't. I figured it was not likely that I could keep my blood pressure completely under control without some medication, but I could reduce the amount of medication I might need by getting physically fit. I could do that by exercising regularly, including some kind of aerobics.

Then I looked at cholesterol. The way my numbers were, I figured it was not likely that I could get off medication entirely to control that either, but again I could reduce what medication I might need to a minimum by getting physically fit.

Then I looked at the diabetes issue. In my research, I figured out that type II diabetes is not really diabetes at all. Not the way I had always understood it. I always understood that diabetes is when your body cannot produce enough insulin to process the sugar you eat. But that's not how type II works. When you have type II diabetes, you may be producing insulin all right, and you might actually be producing a lot of it. But the real problem is that your body just isn't able to use that insulin as well as you could when you were younger.

When you have too much sugar in your blood, your body tries to reduce those sugar levels by storing it somewhere. We all know that it stores it in your cells as fat. But in order for your cells to accept the sugar and store it, it needs to be bound to insulin. So when your body detects high levels of sugar in your blood, you start producing higher levels of insulin so that the insulin can to go find the sugar, pair up with it and then find a cell to store it in.

When the insulin bound sugar encounters a cell, shows the cell it is paired up with insulin and in effect asks the cell if it can come in and stay a while. Well the cell then, in a manner of speaking, opens the door and in effect, says, "Come on in."

But with type II diabetes something a little bit different happens. The insulin still goes out, finds some sugar to pair up with, then goes knocking on doors (cells) to try and find a place to store it. Except now it's kind of like your cells are too tired to open the door to let the sugar-insulin pair in. The solution to this is to load up a lot more insulin in your blood stream. It binds with sugar, but in greater numbers now, so when these sugar-insulin units find a cell, instead of politely knocking and asking if they can come in, this insulin loaded sugar just forces its way into the cell to go into storage. It's kind of like the extra insulin just knocks down the door and forces its way inside.

This does work, because if you have type II diabetes, taking a shot of insulin does reduce your blood sugar levels. But it means you are solving the problem of high sugar levels, by using elevated levels of insulin to force the sugar into the cells. The real root problem is that your cells just aren't working as efficiently as they used to, when you were younger. In this respect they are sort of acting like they are old and tired. That is really the problem. So how do you fix that?

Well one way is to rely on using the extra insulin. That's certainly a lot better than doing nothing about it. Chronic high sugar levels are very damaging to your body in a lot of ways. But that doesn't attack the real problem, and will probably make you get fatter if you're not careful. The other way is to get healthy and get fit, again by vigorous exercise, including aerobics. In talking to my doctor about this, he confirmed that if I could lose weight and exercise regularly, the type II diabetes symptoms I had would likely completely disappear.

As I looked at the other things that my chemistry was telling me, and thought about the diabetes, the high blood pressure, the gooshy plaque just waiting for a good time to rupture again and everything else that had seemed to creep up on me, it appeared that all of my problems would either go away or would be greatly improved if I simply lost weight and started running again. So with my new attitude adjustment, and my urgency to get out of that heart attack danger zone, I decided I would do that. But it was not going to be easy. I had just had a heart attack, I was 310 pounds, and I could not walk a block up a mildly inclined hill, without stopping to rest a bunch of times. It was a tall order to lose a lot of weight and run again.

This is the point where if I was up on a stage talking to a group, or just talking to you one on one, telling you about this, I would say to you that you can do this. I know you can this, because I did it. I am probably more pig headed and stubborn than anyone likely to be reading this book. I spent about twenty years tossing caution to the wind, really knowing I shouldn't do that, but it was just too much to ask to get more control of myself and use a little bit of self-discipline. I even had a good excuse. When I was younger, I learned that I gained weight on the same amount of food others ate who did not gain weight. So I had the perfect excuse to say, I wasn't like other people. I was different. I couldn't do this. But that's sort of like saying, "I have a thyroid problem, so it's not my fault. I can't do anything about it."

I made up my mind that thinking along those lines was just an excuse. I could lose weight if I really wanted to. I would just have to find that level of eating, whatever it was, that was not enough to sustain my 310 pounds. Once I got there, I would have to lose weight. The laws of physics say so. It might be that I would be eating a lot less than most other people, but there would be a point I could find where I had to lose weight. And there would be point where I could maintain a proper weight. It is just not a one size fits all world.

But what about the running? I was much older now, not in my twenties any more. I had just had a heart attack, could I even do that?

I went back to visit my cardiologist about two weeks later. A day or two before the appointment, I had gone in for some blood work, for a battery of chemistry tests and X-rays.

When I sat down, after exchanging pleasantries, he said he had been looking over my test results and was very surprised at what the results showed. He put it this way, in his Russian accent, "You know, if you were to walk into some other doctor's office with these test results, and tell him that you had a heart attack two weeks ago, he would call you a liar."

He went on to explain that when a person has a heart attack, such as the one I had, even in a mild case, there are chemical traces of it in the blood afterward. I had no chemical markers at all and that was quite remarkable. He also told me the detailed X-ray photos they had taken of my heart during the lab work session a couple of days back, likewise showed no signs whatever of any sort of heart event having ever taken place. He went on to say that was quite remarkable as well, because he was there, he saw me, I did have a heart attack, but yet, examining me now, it was as if it never happened.

I felt very lucky at that point and started talking to him about where to go from here. I told him that I wanted to get fit again and asked about exercising and the rest of my plan to eventually start running again. He told me there was nothing standing in my way, and that is what he was going to recommend I do anyway. He said my routine should be to lose weight, and do aerobics every day, from now on. He told me the best approach to the aerobics was to begin by walking, for a minimum of twenty minutes every day. During that walk, a mile or so, I was to walk fast, as fast as I could comfortably do it. He said the goal was to eventually get my heart rate up to about 120, and keep it there for twenty minutes. I was to do that every day.

A couple of days later I went to visit my new family medical doctor. I had much the same conversation with him. After I told him what I wanted to do, he was all for it, and mentioned how few people really take to heart what being fit and exercising does for your general health. We agreed that for most people it's just too much trouble and they don't want to do it. They simply want a pill. We have come a very long way on what those "pills" can do for you. But there is so much you can do for yourself that is even better than just the pills.

Chapter five
Putting My Plan Into Action.

This all happened to me during the month of May, so when I was able to get back to work, it was June. It was nice weather, warm outside, great weather for taking a walk. So that's what I did. I worked on an air force base that was quite spread out, so it was easy to map out a route to walk that would suit my needs.

I mapped out a nice walking route that was about a mile and a half long. Then I started to walk it during lunchtime instead of eating lunch. I noticed there were some other people who walked during lunch as well. There weren't too many of them, but there were a few.

At first, it was a real struggle just to finish this route. It was warm weather, so I did sweat just a bit from the workout. I was just walking, but still, it wasn't easy. But I kept it up for over a month. Sometimes I felt like people were looking at me, thinking I was a walrus out for a stroll.

As for my eating habits, I knew I had to lose weight. But I didn't think it was a good idea to go on one of these fad diets. There are lots of them out there. There are the mail order diets, where they send you food, and you only eat their food. There are diets where you only eat certain things and you lose weight that way. The problem with these diets is that they all come to an end. Some of them do work, and you shed the pounds quickly, but when the diet ends, it ends, you are done, you have lost the weight, so what do you do then? Well since you can't keep doing the diet, you usually go back to your old habits and put the pounds back on.

I had to do something that was going to last. I had to do something that was going to be a way of life. It couldn't be something that I couldn't do after I'd lost the weight. This had to be what was normal for me from now on. The only thing that made sense was to do what I just mapped out. Eat what I needed and not more. Again it sounds simple but it takes discipline.

Food is all around us, just about everywhere. You can't drive down the street without seeing fast food places and restaurants. If you stand in line at the hardware store, there are candy bars and things to tempt you. And it looks like such a small thing, a little candy bar. What harm could that do? They are packed with energy and if you don't use that energy, you get fat. That's the harm.

I ate breakfast, usually something low carb. But I did mix it up with other things like pancakes, and oatmeal. I had a light dinner, heavy on veggies, then, for a late night snack, maybe a small helping of ice cream.

In changing my eating habits, I really didn't do anything other than eat much less. I still ate many of the things I liked, I just didn't eat very much of them or very often. Before my heart attack, I was eating anytime and anywhere I felt like, because I do like food. But you have to understand, that as much as you might like it, too much is not good. So the new mindset I had to adjust to was, food is the enemy. But it is an enemy that you must live with. You cannot banish food from your world. And the worst part is, food does taste good, and I really like it. But I simply had to develop the discipline to decide ahead of time what I was going to eat, how much and when. And it worked. I did begin to lose weight, very slowly, but it was working. This kind of plan was something I could stick to after I'd lost the weight I needed to lose. It simply amounted to being aware of what you are eating, and watch the scale. Then eat less than you need when you need to lose weight.

This sounds pretty simple and it is, unless you start comparing what you are eating to the government guidelines or something. For me, eating three square meals a day will put on about five pounds a week. What you have to do is find out what you need. Go by that and not by what some chart is telling you. If 500 calories a day will work for you. Do that. If it's 5,000 a day, do that. But you need to figure out what you need, and get used to it and live that way.

The key to the discipline part of it for me was to plan what I was going to eat and when I was going to eat it. This might not work for you but it seemed to me that having the day of eating planned out, and not eating anything that was not on the plan really helped.

I am not one who is able to say, "It's time for lunch, let's go find something to eat," without ending up eating too much almost every time. It seemed that everything I found was so good, I wanted another and it seemed like such a small thing, to have just one more. That's where the planning part helped. If you walk into a place and you know exactly what you are going to eat. It helps. It keeps me from looking the menu over to see if there's something better. It's the same when you open your cupboard or refrigerator at home. Never do that, looking or browsing for something to eat. Open it to get something that you know is there and that's what you are going to eat. You are not going to browse. You are going to get it and eat it because it's on your plan and it's time to eat it.

There's not much else to say about my eating, other than it amazed me, how little you really need to eat to stay healthy. I never eat three squares a day any more. I can't because I know that will put the weight back on real fast. Much of the time, I only eat one meal, and it's not a big meal. That's all I need. At first it really bothered me because I was so hungry all the time. But after a while, and it took a while, it didn't bother me anymore. Eating once a day become normal for me, and I really didn't get that hungry in between.

Chapter six
My Recovery Begins

As I continued on the exercise program, the walking got easier. I began losing weight, maybe a pound or sometimes two a week. But if I cheated at all, ate a cookie, or bought a candy bar or did something like that, I could really tell. The weight loss progress stopped for a day or two. Also if I did that, my sugar levels would spike right away and I would have to go inject myself with insulin to bring it back down.

It was encouraging that the weight was coming off and that I was able to walk with less effort, but I was still a long ways off from attempting to jog.

I stayed with this routine for the next year. Some weeks I would lose weight, some I didn't. There were even some weeks I actually gained weight, but I stayed with it. I noticed that the need for insulin shots was not as dramatic now. When I checked my glucose level before and after eating something that would usually spike my sugar levels, the spikes would be less, requiring less insulin. So something was getting better.

After about a year, all of my chemistry levels had dramatically improved. A1C level had actually plummeted to 5.8. I didn't keep it that low all the time, but I did hit it. I was very careful to never let my glucose levels spike above 150. I tried to keep it at about 100 or lower most of the time. I did this by being very careful about what I ate, and monitoring the levels several times a day. As time went on, I noticed that it was taking less and less insulin to manage the glucose spikes. Then sometimes the spikes even began to limit themselves, without the need for any insulin. This was definite progress.

I remember one day, after I had lost about thirty pounds, I decided to try and jog a couple of hundred feet during my daily walk. So I picked up the pace and started jogging, very slowly, but I was doing a slow bouncy jog. It was awful. It felt like my insides were going to tear themselves apart. The bouncing sensation on my organs and belly was pretty bad, nearly painful, but I kept it up for as long as I could, which was only about 150 feet or so. I just couldn't go any further. It was a combination of being out of breath and the trauma of shaking my insides so badly. But this was not a failure. It was a success. I would never have even attempted to do that before the heart attack. But I did jog, even though it was a short distance, I had done it. Now it would be to try and improve on that.

I figured it really wasn't practical to be jogging during my lunchtime walking session because I would get too sweaty and have to take a shower before getting back to work. So jogging at work was out. But since I had showed myself that I could do it now, I needed to figure out some other way to work on the jogging.

I dusted off an old treadmill I had at home in the basement. I can't remember when I bought it, but like most people who buy these things, I had tried to use it a couple of times, but then it became a coat rack. I guess it had been sitting there, unused for four or five years. I plugged it in and fired it up. Good news. It still worked. I checked it over and all seemed to be well.

With a working treadmill, I figured what I would do is walk at the base as usual during lunchtime, but then every day I would get on the treadmill at home in the evening, set it for two miles an hour, and walk that for 30 minutes. During that walk I was going to try and jog for a minute or two at a time, until I got too winded. That was how I figured I could work on building up from there, and hopefully, eventually begin to actually run.

Well I did that for a few months and I did actually get to a point where I was able to jog for about five minutes at a time. At first it was a rather jarring experience, about like the time I tried to jog on the base during my lunchtime walk. But I kept trying and it got better. Over time it got better until the jarring sensation went away.

One thing bad about the treadmill was it was very boring. To pass the time I started listening to audiobooks. Then I started watching movies on a screen I set up in front of me. I was on that treadmill for a half hour, and once this became a routine thing I did every day, the time seemed to crawl by while I was doing it. The movies helped with the boredom and I kept it up.

After about six months of doing this, when I went in for my medical checkups, my chemistry kept improving. The cholesterol was much better, so we reduced the medication I was taking for that. My A1C was still down, and I was using much less insulin.

After about three years, I finally got down to about 240 pounds and I was able to run, not just jog, but actually run, at full speed, which for me was six miles an hour, according to the treadmill. Now that's not Olympic speed, but for a fat old guy like me, that was really good. Running was fun again, and I could do it.

I started to notice some other things that began to happen. My dental checkups turned out better than expected. I had been experiencing receding gums, and the condition had seemed to reverse itself. I didn't think that was possible, but it did. Talking to my dentist about it, he figured it could be due to my body chemistry getting so much better, especially blood sugar levels. He told me that people who are diabetic experience worse problems with their teeth and gums than non-diabetics.

I started paying attention to doing some ordinary things that I dreaded because they were so difficult to do, like crawling under the dashboard of a car to make a repair or under the kitchen sink to fix a drain pipe. This used to be such a pain because it was physically so difficult to do. I was so fat, I guess, that it was just really difficult to get into those positions to work. But now, as I was doing these kinds of jobs, I started to take notice that it wasn't so difficult anymore.

After the two year mark somewhere, I had stopped using the insulin pens entirely. I was still careful about what I ate, not really in what it was I was eating, but just how much. I was more concerned about not gaining weight and not really so concerned about not eating sugar, or fat or things like that. I could now actually eat a big piece of cake, with frosting on it, and not have it spike my sugar levels any more. They would go up, but not much worse than when I was twenty five, taking that glucose tolerance test in the navy, so many years ago.

Chapter seven
I Did It, I won

I have kept this program up for about six years now. My checkups have always been good. My chemistry is always great. I am taking blood pressure and cholesterol medications, but during the process of getting fit, I have reduced the amount of medication I need to maintain my blood pressure and cholesterol levels by a significant degree. I am not really dependent on those. It is more like they give me a degree of extra help, and it's worth it. The last time I went in, my blood pressure was 118/87. My pulse was 48. My A1C was under 7. The rest is the same, very good.

Before the heart attack, my blood pressure was always 160 or 180 over something, with a pulse rate of 80 or so. The dramatic difference is due to the exercise and weight loss more than anything else. I feel better, I am more alert. I don't get sick as much. In short, everything about life that has anything to do with health is much better.

The price I pay for this dramatically improved health is a one hour session of vigorous exercise, including 35 minutes of running the treadmill every other day. That's a bit less than what I was doing at the peak of becoming fit. I am now only trying to maintain fitness because I have gotten there. I am physically fit now. I recall on one visit to my cardiologist, he told me it was okay to back down on the physical exercise program a bit because, "You are not an athlete in training you know. You can back off a bit now. You have done it."

So I did. I have a routine now that I do every other day. It lasts an hour, and like I said, it includes 35 minutes of hard core running. I have actually worn out three treadmill machines now. I have purchased some weights and a rowing machine that have been a regular part of the workout for quite a while now. I have outfitted a "Mancave" to accommodate my workouts, with a large screen entertainment center and a powerful surround sound speaker system that I watch movies on. When I don't feel like watching a movie, I have a few concert DVD's of ZZ TOP, Doobie Brothers, and some others that I put on. I crank it up and watch the concert while I run.

My workouts are really intense now and actually they are fun. I sometimes think back to how it was seven years ago and where I am now. It's a difference of day and night. I have far exceeded what even my doctors had expected. I went hiking in the mountains last summer with some younger family members. I had to stop and take a break several times, to let them catch up to me. Life is good. Life is better when you are physically fit, especially when you are passing middle age.

You can do this too. I am 63 years old now. I am fit and in excellent health. It was only about 7 years ago; I was on an operating table, lucky that I had made it to the hospital in time.

The choice is yours. You can do this too. Don't end up getting a heart attack like I did. Unless you have a condition or congenital problem that actually prevents you from exercising, there is no reason you can't do this.

It's not easy doing this. It takes time. It takes patience. At times, it has been painful getting to this point. But I am here, and it was worth it. It is worth it to keep doing this. I have made up my mind that I am going to extend my healthy life as long as I can. This way of life is going to help me do that. I am not going to die, after several years in a rest home, in a wheel chair, with drool running out of my mouth. I am going to die on that treadmill, on my feet.

I will sustain my good life much longer on the treadmill than without it. And those will be good years.

Chapter eight
Last Word

If you are middle aged, getting to your fifties or more. Don't wait until you have a heart attack. You might not be as lucky as I was. Keep your weight under control and exercise regularly, including a good set of aerobics for your heart. Find a good doctor and get regular checkups. Watch your chemistry. Learn what the chemistry means. Do these things and you will stay healthy and on your feet longer. Life will be better.